CW00739423

Leslie Kenton is an award-winning writer, novelist, teacher, social activist and bestselling author of more than thirty books. A well-known TV broadcaster and the daughter of jazz musician Stan Kenton, Leslie has spent more than twenty-five years working in the realms of health, philosophy and the exploration of consciousness. She first became famous for books such as *Raw Energy* and *Ageless Ageing*, which have been translated into many languages. For fourteen years she was an editor for *Harpers & Queen*.

Author's Note

The material in this book is intended for information purposes only. None of the suggestions or information is meant in any way to be prescriptive. Any attempt to treat a medical condition should always come under the direction of a competent medical practitioners – and neither the publisher nor I can accept responsibility for injuries or illness arising out of a failure by a reader to take medical advice. I am only a reporter. I also have a profound interest in helping myself and others to maximise our potential for positive health which includes being able to live at a high level of energy, intelligence and creativity. For all three are expressions of harmony within a living organic system.

Leslie Kenton
KICK COLDS

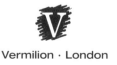

Vermilion · London

First published in the United Kingdom in 2000 by Vermilion, an imprint of Random House
20 Vauxhall Bridge Road · London SW1V 2SA

Random House Australia (Pty) Limited
20 Alfred Street · Milsons Point · Sydney · New South Wales 2061 · Australia

Random House New Zealand Limited
18 Poland Road · Glenfield · Auckland 10 · New Zealand

Random House South Africa (Pty) Limited
Endulini · 5a Jubilee Road · Parktown 2193 · South Africa

Random House Group Limited Reg. No. 954009

A CIP catalogue record for this book is available from the British Library

ISBN: 0 09 182583 0

Designed by Lovelock & Co.

Printed and bound by Sheck Wah Tong Printing Press Ltd

CONTENTS

1 INSTANT HELP

One of the most frustrating and persistent illnesses is the common cold. It can be a pain in the neck, in the head and sometimes even in the bottom, too. But this doesn't mean you have to sit back and take everything a cold can throw at you. There are lots of things you can do at the first sign of symptoms to keep it from taking hold and dragging you down. I believe no-one need ever suffer a full-blown attack again. You just need to know about natural treatments and prevention.

Colds can hit fast: you wake up one morning with a hot feeling at the back of your nose, a scratchy throat and eyes that are too big for their sockets. This is the moment to act. You come down with a cold for two reasons: your body needs to eliminate the wastes and toxins it has been carrying around, and your immune system needs a boost. Don't even wait for the first sneeze. Hit hard now.

Go for Herbs

Reach immediately for tincture of echinacea. This immune-enhancing plant in liquid form acts quickly (more quickly than taking capsules) to get your whole system buzzing. Take a teaspoon in water every hour or two for the first day. Then 1–2 teaspoons three or four times a day until the symptoms have gone.

Get into C

Take 6–10 g of vitamin C at regular intervals throughout the day, each day, until your cold has cleared. Because it is water soluble, vitamin C is not stored in the tissues. Once your tissues have been saturated, any excess is excreted in the urine.

Taking vitamin C in quantities greater than the body can use will cause loose bowels. Robert Cathcart, an American physician known throughout the world for his work with vitamin C, believes this can offer a good indication of just how much vitamin C you need at any time, whether you are ill or not. He uses doses of the vitamin ranging from 10 g to 200 g a day given orally to treat serious illness. The appropriate dose for any individual, he says, is just below the point at which the bowels become loose.

As soon as a cold hits, I take 6 g of vitamin C a day. This is an average dose for an average person with a cold. If your bowels become loose then cut back a little on this dose. If you feel you need more vitamin C, increase the dose until your bowels loosen, then cut back a little.

Tea Off

Have a hot cup of tea – herb tea, not your ordinary caffeine-rich black tea – to get your circulation going. If your blood is moving smoothly around your body it will be able to clear infection from your system that much more quickly. Make your tea from something you have to hand, don't wait until you get a chance to shop. Good herb teas for colds include ginger, yarrow, peppermint, elderflower, camomile, lemon balm, lemon verbena, sage, thyme, rosemary or basil. Steep 1 teaspoon (or a teabag if that's what you have) of the dried herb in a cup of boiling water for 5–10 minutes. Use 2 teaspoons of the fresh leaves or flowers if you have them. Take a cup of soothing white willow tea if you have a headache. If you like your tea sweet then add a good dollop of honey. It has anti-bacterial properties that will help with your cold, too.

Zap with Zinc

Researchers have found that the most effective way of taking zinc for colds is in the form of a lozenge which is allowed to dissolve in the mouth. I find that sucking on a zinc lozenge can instantly relieve a tickly throat.

Get Garlicky

Garlic is nature's antibiotic. Put an unpeeled clove of garlic in your cheek – tuck it between your cheek and bottom teeth or jaw – and leave it there for half an hour or so. The garlic will instantly get to work killing off any bugs in your mouth and throat, and will cure a sore throat quicker than anything else I have found.

Take a Bath

Get straight into an Epsom-salts bath. In fact, run your bath while your herb tea is brewing and drink it while you are enjoying your bath. Epsom salts are magnesium sulphate. Both magnesium and sulphate molecules have an ability to leach excess sodium, phosphorus and nitrogenous wastes from the body. During a cold your body is going through a process of throwing off wastes while it tries to eliminate infection. An Epsom-salts bath will help with this process and will also relieve any muscular aches and pains that have come with your cold.

Take two cups of household-grade Epsom salts (available from the chemist), pour it into the bath and fill the bath with blood-heat water. Then immerse yourself for twenty–thirty minutes, topping up with warm water when necessary to maintain a comfortable temperature. Afterwards, lie down for fifteen minutes.

Lie Back

Don't try to go to work. You could simply be spreading your illness around. You might get Brownie points for turning up, but you'll lose them all again when everyone else goes off sick. Allowing yourself to rest while you have a cold gives your body the chance to concentrate on getting well. Wrap yourself up warmly, and stay put until you have conquered your cold.

Go Raw

Stop eating convenience foods and read the next chapter which contains all the information you need to put paid to a cold.

2 TO EAT OR NOT TO EAT

When a cold strikes, your body is looking for an excuse to detoxify itself. Go with the flow and help your system with its elimination processes. You will often feel far better after your cold is over than you did before it began.

Cut the Junk

While your body is doing its stuff in clearing out all the rubbish it has accumulated over weeks, months, even years, you don't want to be putting yet more in. Cut out convenience foods and avoid all wheat products. Stop drinking tea and coffee. The caffeine in them is too stimulating. It's particularly important to avoid milk products like yoghurt, cheese, cream and milk itself as well as anything containing them. Milk products are highly mucus-forming and will only make your runny nose or blocked sinuses worse. The mucus that comes with a cold actually consists of dead white blood cells which have done their job fighting off infection. You don't want slow down the system by giving your body even more mucus to process.

Also avoid sugar. Too much sugar undermines the power of white blood cells so they are less able to fight infection. It also interferes with your body's uptake of vitamin C, which you really want to make the most of during a cold.

In the Raw

At the first sign of a cold or flu I go raw. Raw foods have remarkable cleansing and healing properties.

When you are ill your body is burning up wastes and fighting off an invasion. It doesn't need to cope with digesting heavy meals too. Uncooked foods such as fresh crisp vegetables, luscious fruits and natural unprocessed seeds, grains and nuts have a quality of energy which is light yet strong and extraordinarily health-giving. Such foods are the richest natural sources of vitamins, minerals and enzymes, as well as fine-quality protein, easily assimilated natural carbohydrates and essential fatty acids. They are also an excellent source of unadulterated natural fibre, and put no strain on your digestive system.

Fruit Freedom

At the first sign of a cold the best way to kick-start the whole elimination process is to eat fruit – and only one kind of fruit as this puts the least stress on your digestive system. Apples or grapes are excellent. The high fibre content of apples also makes them great intestinal 'brooms'.

Grapes are very effective cleansers due to their potent properties which counter excessive mucus. Grapes provide a quick source of energy which helps when a cold has made you feel low and sluggish.

How much fruit you choose to eat depends on how you feel. You may need to eat it more frequently than usual as fruit is digested very quickly and does not remain in the stomach for more than an hour. You might want to take about four or five fruit meals at intervals throughout the day (eating continually is tiring for the digestive system), but don't go hungry. If you get bored, try grating your apples into a bowl and sprinkling a little cinnamon over them, or blend them with a little crushed ice to make a fruit frappe. Grapes are a bit more restricting in that there isn't a lot you can do with them, but there are all sorts of interesting ways you can try to eat them – such as tossing them up in the air and catching them in your mouth.

Go Easy

Until your cold has completely cleared up, continue to support the elimination process but bring in other raw fruits and vegetables to nourish and rebalance your system. Begin the day with fruit for breakfast. The liver – the organ of detoxification – is at its most active in the morning so you don't want to give it too much to do. Have a salad or another fruit meal for lunch. For your evening meal make yourself a large raw salad and toss in a few sunflower seeds or almonds and season with fresh herbs.

Once your cold has cleared, ease gently back into eating three full meals a day. Stay with the fruit breakfast for a few days, have your salad for lunch, and steam or lightly wok-fry some vegetables for your evening meal. Gradually over three or four days introduce the odd bowl of soup, piece of steamed or grilled fish, chicken, or side-serving of brown rice or millet.

You may find that this way of eating suits you so well that you don't want to go back to eating convenience foods and drinking coffee. But more of this later when we look at how to protect yourself from getting colds in the future.

Walk it Off

Gentle exercise also helps with detoxification. But I mean gentle. When your body starts throwing off wastes like this it needs all the energy you can give it. Don't squander it by going for a run. Try easy walks in the fresh air and take plenty of deep breaths. Your lungs are important waste eliminators, gathering up toxins and expelling them with every out breath. Try breathing in deeply to a count of 10, then hold your breath for a count of 20, exhale to a count of 10 and hold it for a count of 10. This will help to make your nose, throat and head feel clearer and will get your blood moving through your whole body mopping up toxins and flushing them out.

And make sure you get plenty of rest. We'll look at that next.

3 TAKE COMFORT

Two things heal a cold. Nutrition (food, water, herbs and supplements) and rest. Allowing yourself to rest while you have a cold gives your body the chance to concentrate on getting well. If you carry on working, you are using up energy that could be put to good use by your body elsewhere. You know yourself just how hard it is to concentrate when you have a cold so if you feel you really have to keep working then at least slow down.

Your best bet is to wrap yourself up and stay on the sofa. Better still, go to bed. Your body is taking this opportunity to rid itself of toxins, but it is also telling you to get some rest. How many times have we cursed a cold for coming at just the wrong time? Or gone down with one at the end of a really stressful time at work? Your body is telling you that you need to slow down. Take heed or it might just throw something worse at you.

The Heat is On

The first thing to remember is to keep warm. Your immune system has enough to do without worrying about keeping your temperature up. If you feel hot, don't fight it. Raising your temperature is one of your body's defence mechanisms. White blood cells signal the brain to raise the body's temperature to kill off bacteria and viruses which on the whole prefer things to be cool. If your fever goes higher than 40°C (104°F), however, see your doctor.

The archetypal image of a cold victim is someone sitting in a chair with his or her feet in a bowl of steaming water. Old-fashioned as it may seem, a hot foot bath is actually one of the most useful techniques for treating colds. It brings on sweating which is another of the body's ways of getting rid of toxins, helps with congestion and relieves headaches.

You can immerse your feet up to the ankles in hot water for about fifteen minutes. Keep topping the bowl up with hot water so that it remains as hot as you can stand it, and keep the rest of your body well wrapped up. After fifteen minutes rinse your feet quickly with cold water, dry them well and wrap them in warm socks.

Bathe it Away

A long, hot soak can do a lot to bring equilibrium to a mind and body wracked by a cold. Keep the water topped up and hot. An Epsom-salts bath (see page 10) will help with any aches and pains. Adding two–three drops of a good-quality essential oil and breathing them in with the steam can help you to deal with the other inconveniences that can come with a cold. Try:

Cold Essentials

TO CHEER YOU UP	Hyssop, marjoram, sandalwood
TO EASE WORRY	Lavender
TO MAKE YOU FEEL STRONGER	Camomile, jasmine, melissa
TO SOOTHE IRRITABILITY	Frankincense, marjoram, camomile, lavender
TO RELIEVE EXHAUSTION	Jasmine, rosemary, juniper, patchouli
TO UNKNOT ANXIETY	Sage, juniper, basil, jasmine

Treat Yourself

If you're feeling really miserable, then treat yourself to a hot toddy. No more than one a day, though, as you want to give your digestion as little to do as possible. Have one just before bed to help you to get to sleep.

'Hot' aromatic spices are great for a cold: ginger, cinnamon, cloves and coriander seeds. Put a cup of red wine in a saucepan and drop in a couple of whole cloves, a pinch of powdered cinnamon, a pinch of powdered ginger, and a few crushed coriander seeds. Simmer gently for fifteen minutes, strain and drink piping hot.

Grin and Bear It

Doctors and psychologists now acknowledge that your emotional state can contribute to many illnesses. It has now been scientifically proven that a good laugh can do more for your health than just about anything else. Research psychiatrist William Fry, who has been investigating the effect of humour on the body for more than thirty years, has discovered that three minutes of laughter a day is equal to ten minutes of hard aerobic exercise. (It probably took him thirty years to work it out because he was having so much fun.) Laughter benefits the heart, increases the body's use of oxygen, reduces muscle tension, pulse rate and blood pressure. It also has a marvellously stimulating effect on the immune system. Depressed people usually have depressed immunity, too. In simple terms, the happier you are and the better you feel about yourself, the less likely you are to fall prey to illnesses of any sort.

So while you are wrapped up on the sofa with a red nose and your feet are in a bowl of steaming water, have a good laugh at how ridiculous you look. Better still, watch some of your favourite funny films on video and read a humorous book or two. You'll probably feel much better straight away.

4 DRINK LIKE A FISH

Colds make things dry. That's why you often get a dry throat and sore chest along with the coughing and sneezing. Drinking lots of fluids keeps everything lubricated and kick starts your body's elimination of wastes. However, the myth that you need glass after glass of orange juice to fight a cold is simply untrue. Packaged orange juices are low in vitamin C and high in sugar which will inhibit your immune system and put extra strain on your digestion. If you want the vitamin C, then take it as a supplement. Help to get rid of a cold fast by supporting your body's waste-disposal effort: drink water. Lots of it.

Water Wonders

Water is the most important nutrient of all. It is the stuff from which your blood, your cells, your muscles – even your bones – are mostly made. A healthy person who weights 65 kilos (11 stone) carries about 40 litres (70 pints) of water around – 25 litres (45 pints) inside the cells, 15 litres (28 pints) outside, including 5 litres (9 pints) in the blood. If you let yourself become dehydrated, chemical reactions in your cells become sluggish and toxic products build up in your bloodstream.

The brain too is seventy-five per cent water. This is why the quantity and quality of water you drink affects how you think and feel. Water is vital during a cold to counteract the feelings of low energy and muzzy-headedness. But if the water you drink is polluted by heavy metals or chemicals then you will become polluted as well. Watch what you drink.

On average, in a temperate climate – not sweating from exertion or heat – we need about 3 litres (five pints) a day for optimum health and to make us resistant to colds, although few of us consume even as much as one litre (2 pints). The important thing to remember is that your level of thirst is not a reliable indication of how much water you need to drink. Here's how to work out your own daily water needs:

Divide your current weight in kilos by 8. If you weigh 58 kilos then 58 divided by 8 equals 7.25 big glasses. Then round the figure up and there you have it: eight glasses a day. But remember that is only a base calculation for when you are well. *You will need to drink more than this when you have a cold.*

Only Water Works

What about other drinks – coffee and tea, soft drinks and fruit juices? Won't they do just as well? No they won't. Quite apart from the other negative effects of caffeine – an ingredient in coffee, tea and many soft drinks – drinking coffee messes up your blood sugar. Caffeine is a habit-forming drug. It has frequently been shown to be responsible for headache, insomnia, nervousness, anxiety, and that familiar wired mental state which gets you buzzing for a time. Caffeine gives you a quick lift and the illusion of energy only to let you crash down a couple of hours later, making you inclined to reach for more – or for a sticky bun or chocolate – just to keep going.

Coffee also tends to raise blood pressure and to increase the risk of coronary thrombosis. Drink five cups each day and your heart-attack risk goes up by sixty per cent.

What about tea? It too contains caffeine – 100 mg to coffee's 120 mg in a regular-sized cup. Tea also contains tannic acid, an irritant to the digestive system. Even if you have always been a committed six to eight cups a day tea or coffee drinker, after a couple of weeks on good water you will find you don't miss it. Then when you have an occasional cup it becomes a simple pleasure rather than an addiction.

Cut the Soft Drinks

The average intake of soft drinks in the West has risen to eight to twelve a week in some countries – between 400 and 600 a year. Many colas, squashes and soft drinks also contain caffeine. And they are also far too high in sugar. A small can of cola contains seven teaspoons of sugar – about 40 g. It is full of chemicals which pollute your body and overload your body's elimination processes.

Fruit juices are OK but remember that they are highly concentrated in sugar. It takes between three to five oranges to make a glass of juice. So far so good if you drink only one glass but bear in mind that you would not eat all those oranges in one go. Water puts a lot less stress on your system when you have a cold.

Herb teas such as peppermint, camomile, vervain and lemon grass are also OK. By all means drink them and enjoy them. But stay away from the fancy packaged ones unless you read the labels carefully and make sure they are entirely natural. Many contain artificial flavours or calories which you don't need. But don't count them into your daily water quota. Think of them as extras. The bottom line is simple: water is best by far. The only problem these days is how to find water that is fit to drink.

Drink Your Health

Bottled waters vary tremendously. Some are nothing more than tap water which has been run through conditioning filters to remove the taste while doing nothing to improve the quality. And just because they say 'spring' on the label doesn't mean a thing. The word may be nothing more than the brand name used to sell the product. Other bottled waters are excellent in taste and quality. Few countries do much to regulate standards for bottled water. Except France.

There are some 1,200 springs in France. Several dozen of

them supply bottled waters the quality of which has long been monitored and controlled by official government bodies. These waters should be safe from bacterial or chemical contamination and you can be sure they have not been mixed with any foreign substance when they are bottled.

Get Drinking

Provided you have no kidney disease or other condition which would mean your doctor would disapprove, whatever water you choose to drink, start now to drink a lot of it and keep drinking a lot of it after you have got over your cold. As long as your kidneys are normal you need not worry about drinking too much. But drink your water between meals, not with them. Water drunk with meals dilutes the potency of digestive juices needed to properly break down and assimilate nutrients from your food.

It takes a bit of practice at first to make sure you get your water quota each day but soon it will become second nature. Start by drinking two glasses of water first thing in the morning, either neat or with a twist of lemon or lime. You can heat the water if you like to help with elimination. Then drink two or three glasses between breakfast and lunch and another two or three between lunch and dinner. Keep a bottle or two of mineral water by you during the day as an easy measure of just how much you need to drink to get your daily quota. Each time you visit the toilet (you will do this a lot more frequently when you first start your water-drinking), give thanks for the deep cleansing which is taking place – clearing away your cold in the process.

5 PROTECT AND SURVIVE

Knowing how to deal with a cold when one strikes is only half the story. Learn a few simple rules and make use of a few helpers and you can protect yourself so well that you may never suffer a cold again. As we have seen, there are two reasons why you get a cold in the first place: your body needs to clear out wastes and toxins; and your immune system needs some help. Let's look at immunity first.

Colds are associated with up to 200 viruses. Viruses are so small that you can't even see them under a normal microscope. Scientists can't decide if they are living things or not since they don't eat, use oxygen, or eliminate wastes. What they do is to reproduce inside your body. Anti-viral drugs are as scarce as hen's teeth, and antibiotics can't deal with viruses. But your immune system can. A fit and healthy immune system is the key to freedom from just about any illness, so don't let yours become slack and lazy.

Secret Police

Your immune system is a complex network of specialised cells and processes which form your body's natural defence against invasion, poison and disease.

There are two sides to immunity: the secret police – the

Leslie's Immune Boosters

- Take between 1 and 3g of vitamin C a day
- Take a good multi-vitamin and mineral supplement every day
- Drink three cups of astragalus tea a day
- Eat plenty of fresh garlic
- Include immune-stimulating Japanese mushrooms in your cooking

---

humoral immunity; and the militia – the cell-mediated immunity. Your humoral immunity collects a vast log of thousands of antibodies which it has created in response to specific viruses, chemicals, bacteria and foreign substances which have invaded your system throughout your lifetime. When your body is invaded by a new one, it is the militia, the cell-mediated immunity, which goes out to fight it. This part of your immune system is centred around specialised cells called T-cell and B-cell lymphocytes. Build it up and you have an in-built resistance to infection.

C Your Army

An army marches on its stomach, they say. You can keep your immune system's army well-fed by giving it some extra nutritional support, beginning with vitamin C. When T-cells set about killing infection they need lots of vitamin C and mop up all that they can find in your system like little sponges. Even when they are not out fighting, T-cells contain a high concentration of vitamin C. Ageing, illness, smoking, and stress all cause the levels of vitamin C in your body to drop, so lowering the ability of the T-cells to do their job properly.

Taking preventative doses of vitamin C will help to keep your T-cells in peak fighting condition.

Nutrient Know-How

Many of the B-complex vitamins such as vitamin B1, B2, B3, B6, pantothenic acid, B12, and folic acid are also particularly important in maintaining a sturdy immune system. So is the element chromium. And vitamin E has also been shown in many studies to boost resistance to illness. People with high levels of vitamin E get significantly fewer infections than those with average levels. Beta-carotene (from which your body can make vitamin A) has also been shown to increase the response of natural killer-cells to immune challenges, and vitamin A increases the size of the thymus gland – the gland which directs the actions of the immune system. The minerals zinc and selenium are also important to the immune system; zinc deficiency will bring about a rapid decline in the efficiency of T-cell function.

For protection from colds and flu take a good all-round vitamin and mineral supplement, but don't get into the habit of thinking that taking vitamin supplements will make up for a poor diet. It won't.

Sweet Protection

Astragalus is the root of the yellow vetch plant. Unlike many herbs, it actually tastes good. Astragalus brings deep strength to the immune system, increasing the number and quality of white blood cells used to fight infection. Astragalus is an adaptogen, a plant which is often called a 'medicine for well

---

Astragalus Tea

I make enough for three or four cups at a time. This recipe can make a sweet chilled drink but I prefer to reheat mine and drink it warm.

Put six sticks of astragalus, three pieces of liquorice root sticks and a 5-cm (2-in) piece of fresh ginger, peeled and sliced thinly, into a saucepan (not aluminium or non-stick). Pour 1½ litres (just over 2½ pints) of cold water over the herbs and bring the mixture to the boil. Reduce the heat and simmer for twenty minutes. Take it off the heat and allow to stand for ten minutes. Strain and keep in the fridge.

---

people' that, taken over time, will bring strength and support to the whole body.

Three cups of astragalus tea a day helps to ward off colds and flu, as long as you take it consistently every day during the 'cold' season. Chinese medicine defines ailments as being either 'hot' or 'cold' and herbs as being 'warming' or 'cooling'. Astragalus is a 'warming' herb to be used with 'cold' illness, and unless you know what kind of cold or flu you have it is best not to take it while you are unwell. Use it for protection and also as an immune booster after any bout of cold or flu.

Organic astragalus is increasingly available in herb stores dried and shredded. In Chinese pharmacies and Asian markets dried astragalus root looks like ice-lolly sticks. It is cheap and simple to prepare and it makes a mild, sweet tea. Look for sticks which are long and thick, firm yet bendable with a few striations. They should have a sweet taste when you chew on them.

Glorious Garlic

Hundreds of studies have demonstrated garlic's anti-microbial power. It kills bacteria, viruses, fungi and protozoa. It has 5,000 years of recorded history of use against illness. Most things that antibiotic drugs can do, garlic can do better, more safely and cheaper.

Buy your garlic fresh, juiced, in tablets, capsules and tinctures. There are plenty of garlic products which don't give off the characteristic odour if you can't handle it. Garlic acts as a blood thinner so it is wise not to take it with anticoagulant drugs. Taking large daily doses of more than 10 g can cause stomach irritation or indigestion. It is most effective eaten raw and is really enjoyable crushed or minced in salads or on pasta. If you worry about the smell, chew a sprig of parsley after your meal, and never drink cheap red wine with it. It sours the breath badly. Come to think of it, never drink cheap red wine at all. Eat one or two cloves (not bulbs!) of garlic every day in your food.

Listen to the Japanese

Shiitake and Maitake mushrooms not only taste delicious, they contain excellent immune-strengthening compounds, among them the compound lentinan. This phytochemical helps to lower elevated cholesterol. You can take shiitaki and maitake in capsules or as extracts, but I prefer eating the mushrooms themselves. I soak the dried mushrooms and put them in soups and stews and stir-fries.

All of these will help you to ward off colds if you make them a part of your daily life. You won't get their full benefits, however, unless you support your body with a good supply of the nutrients it needs for good health. We'll look at how to do this long-term in the next chapter.

6 EAT FOR RESISTANCE

Colds are your body's way of getting rid of all the wastes and toxins it has collected from our modern life filled with convenience foods, stress, inactivity and pollution. Keep your body free of toxins and you need never have to suffer a cold again. You don't have to live in a plastic bubble and eat like a rabbit. It's common sense. Eat foods that support your body's own ability to clear waste out day by day, and avoid eating foods that put more toxins in.

Shun Convenience Foods

Ready-in-a-minute pre-cooked meals, junk foods and even the standard meat-and-two veg Western meal all fill your body with toxic waste. They present your digestive system with a concentrated protein (e.g., meat) eaten together with a concentrated starch (e.g., bread or potatoes), which are most difficult to break down. Convenience foods and junk foods are also grossly deficient in essential nutrients, further inhibiting your body's ability to eliminate waste.

Most people's bodies cannot efficiently digest more than one concentrated food in the stomach at the same time. In the simplest terms you need an acid medium to digest protein, and an alkaline one to digest starch. If you eat concentrated proteins and starches together (fish and chips, bacon sandwiches, meat and potatoes) neither is properly digested. An awareness of this principle of conscientious food combining lies at the basis of virtually every tradition of natural healing.

If you want to protect your system from a build-up of acid wastes, then begin to separate your concentrated starches from your concentrated proteins, eating each at separate meals.

Back to Nature

For an abundance of energy, it is a good idea not only to separate concentrated proteins from concentrated carbohydrates, but also to be conscientious about what you eat.

Our bodies are not genetically equipped to handle the refined flours, sugars, huge quantities of protein and high concentrations of fat which make up the standard Western fare. Our ancestors did not eat massive quantities of white bread, white sugar, junk fats and pre-packaged, pre-cooked foods. They ate simple, ordinary, wholesome foods – as much of them as they could get.

This way of eating is based on what I call real foods – leafy and root vegetables, whole grains such as brown rice, rye, barley, millet, some pulses, fruits and flesh foods. These foods are naturally low in fat, refined starches and sugars, moderate in protein, rich in fibre, and high in complex carbohydrates. Vegetables and sprouted seeds and grains offer the highest complement of vitamins and minerals, essential fatty acids, easily assimilated top-quality protein, fibre and wholesome carbohydrates found in nature.

Eat Raw

To get the best cold protection from food combining, you need three to four meals a day of which between half and three-quarters should be foods with a naturally high water content (like fresh fruits and vegetables) rather than foods from which moisture has been removed through drying, baking, cooking and processing.

Fresh, uncooked fruits, vegetables, sprouted seeds and sprouted grains all contain high levels of a special kind of water – the water found naturally in living cells. This water is invaluable for helping your body to transport nutrients to all your cells and for taking toxic waste away. This living water is quite different from the stuff that comes out of the tap: water in fresh foods carries electrolytes, vitamins, organic minerals, proteins, enzymes, amino acids, carbohydrates, natural sugars, fatty acids and other nutrients which help to boost cell metabolism.

The remainder of your diet should consist of the stamina-enhancing whole grains, vegetables, legumes, eggs, soya foods like tofu and soya milk, fresh fish, meat, poultry or game. Once you have gained all the energy you want, you can increase your intake of these heavier foods, although many people find that keeping stamina foods to around a third of their diet keeps them feeling and looking well permanently.

Get into Food Combining

Hundreds of years of conventional and complementary medical experience has shown that eating a diet high in raw ingredients, while avoiding certain 'poor' combinations of foods, assists digestion and detoxification. So how does it work? It is based on ten very simple rules that once learned and applied on a daily basis will soon give you a new vitality that comes from a clean and well-nourished system. You need no will-power, you simply follow a healthy diet. The plan is designed to ensure that the food you eat is digested as thoroughly as possible, creating the minimum amount of toxic by-products.

Ten Keys to Clean Living

1 Never eat a concentrated starch food with a concentrated protein food at the same meal. To find out which foods fall into these categories, look at the diagram on pages 46–47. To make sure your diet is balanced, try to eat one carbohydrate-based and one protein-based meal a day.

2 Breakfast should always consist of only fruit or raw vegetables. Your liver is at its most efficient between

midnight and midday. Eating only fruit or drinking fruit or vegetable juice for the first half of the day allows the liver to carry on cleansing at its optimum rate. Eating fruit or drinking fruit juices with other foods can lead to fermentation in the gut causing indigestion and wind. So if later in the day you want to eat fruit with other foods then eat it as a starter rather than a dessert and leave twenty minutes between eating fruit and anything else.

3 Eat a large, raw salad at least once a day. This is the best possible way of enabling your body to rebalance and rebuild itself, restoring metabolism to its peak level.

4 Choose high-quality food. Always make sure that you buy the freshest foods and choose whole-grain, unprocessed varieties of everything whenever possible.

5 Make staples your side dishes. Staple foods include meat, poultry, dairy products, fish, legumes, whole grains and cooked vegetables. They are delicious and satisfying but use them in moderation. The best way to do this is to serve them as side dishes: think of them as condiments to your raw salads and vegetable meals.

6 Eat lots of 'high water' foods. Your body is seventy per cent water. For it to detoxify itself properly, fifty–seventy-five per cent of your daily diet needs to be made up of high-water foods – fresh fruit and vegetables – eaten raw. This is probably one of the easiest guidelines to keep. If you are having only fruit for breakfast and at least one big salad a day, it just about takes care of itself. If you find that you have eaten more staple foods than you should have on any particular day, try to eat nothing but raw foods on the following day to compensate.

7 Don't eat between meals. If you are truly hungry have a piece of fruit or some crunchy raw vegetables. Your system must have time to complete the digestion of a meal before you put anything else into it. Four or five hours need to elapse between lunch and dinner, otherwise digestion will be incomplete which can cause toxicity.

8 Drink plenty of water. Avoid coffee, tea, fizzy drinks and alcohol. They are all high in toxins. Instead, drink plenty of filtered or mineral water and take advantage of the huge number of delicious herb teas available.

9 Be creative. Have fun working out how to put your meals together. It's not difficult and the food is delicious.

10 Make time for exercise. No matter what mountains you have to move to do it, make sure that you set aside time and space to do at least thirty minutes of exercise four times a week. Try some brisk walking, cycling or swimming – anything that gets your heart rate up. Regular exercise spurs the release of toxicity and boosts the metabolism.

Feel Better

If your first response to all this is to say 'How ridiculous, I've been eating meat and potatoes for years and they've never done me any harm!' think about how many colds you've had in your life. By the way, always consult your doctor before undertaking a change in diet if you think you may have a health problem of any kind.

The digestive system of a person who lives on refined foods or who chronically overeats simply doesn't function normally because it remains in a state of permanent stimulation. Many people in this state go on to experience chronic fatigue or hunger and food cravings as the body calls out for the essential vitamins and minerals it is lacking. Poor digestion triggers metabolic slow-down, you lose energy, gain weight easily, and get frequent minor illnesses such as colds and flu.

Don't dismiss food combining as difficult or faddy. It is ridiculously easy, even in a restaurant or at a dinner party. You don't have to clear your plate, whatever your mother told you. In a restaurant, order only what you want or refuse what you don't want when they come to serve the vegetables. At a dinner party it's easy enough to guess that your hosts are probably going to give you protein of some sort, so eat your carbohydrate meal for lunch. Then at dinner just leave what you don't want to eat on your plate.

The all-round benefits of eating this way will amaze you. You won't just find you are free of colds and minor illnesses, you'll also find excess weight falls away and you are full of energy. This is enough of an incentive to keep combining your foods properly, and soon it will be so second nature you won't even think about it.

Conscientious Food-Combining Chart

COMBINATIONS

▨ Poor
Fruit & Starch
Protein & Starch

▨ Fair
Leafy greens & Acid fruits
Leafy greens & Sub-acid fruit
Protein & Acid fruits

▨ Good
Avocado & Acid or Sub-acid fruit
Avocado & Leafy vegetables
Protein & Leafy greens
Starch & Vegetables
Oils & Leafy greens
Oils & Acid or Sub-acid fruits

Starches
Potatoes
Beans and Pulses (Adzuki beans,
Chickpeas, Mung beans,
Lentils, Butter beans, etc.)
Grains (Rice, Wheat, Oats, etc.)
Sweet Potatoes, Pumpkins, etc.

Poor

Proteins
Nuts (Almonds, Cashews, Pecans,
Brazils, Hazelnuts, Walnuts, etc.)
Seeds (Pumpkin, Sunflower,
Sesame, etc.)
Dairy Products – Eggs
Game, Fish, Shellfish, Poultry, etc.

Recommendedations

Make meals of one or two combinations, especially of
one protein or one starch with one or two vegetables

All juices can be mixed because they are liquid and can
be absorbed by the body within half an hour

Neutral foods

(they go well with anything)
Avocado, Olives, Seed oils

Melons

Eat only on their own or leave alone.

Poor

Vegetables

Asparagus, Aubergine, Beetroot, Cabbage, Carrot (mildly starchy), Cucumber, Herbs, Leafy greens, Mustard and cress, Onions, Parsnip, Peas, Salad vegetables, Summer squash, Sweetcorn, Sweet pepper, Turnip, Watercress, Most sprouted seeds and grains etc.

Sweet fruit

Banana, Dates, Dried figs, Persimmon, Raisins and other dried fruit etc.

Fair

Sub-acid fruits

Apple, Apricot, Blackcurrants, Fresh figs, Grapes, Kiwi fruit, Mango, Nectarine, Papaya, Peach, Pear, Sweet Cherries etc.

Good

Acid fruits

Blackberries, Grapefruit, Lemon, Lime, Orange, Pineapple, Plum, Pomegranate, Satsuma, Strawberries, Tangerine, etc.

Fair

Fair

Poor

Fair

od

od

7 FOOD COMBINING FUN

Here are some ideas and suggestions for putting together meals using the principles of conscientious food combining. See how easy it can be.

Fruit or Vegetable Breakfasts

A simple and essential part of the day, your breakfast should consist of nothing but fresh fruit or fresh raw vegetables. They are best eaten like this, on an empty stomach, as their vitamins and minerals are absorbed into the bloodstream almost immediately.

- Eat as much as you like – up to ½ kilo (1lb) at a time – but make sure you chew it thoroughly.

- If you get hungry mid-morning have another piece or two of fruit.
- Eat bananas only if they are very ripe and you feel that you need a heavier food. Do not eat anything else for forty-five minutes.
- Forget fruit and eat only vegetables if you have a blood-sugar or candida problem.
- Never over-eat – but likewise never under-eat. Have as much as you need to feel satisfied. You could try one of these fruit recipes, which can also be eaten as a light supper or energising lunch:

Pear Supreme: Slice four unpeeled pears and lay the slices out in a dish. Mix together two tablespoons of runny honey, the juice of two lemons and three drops of oil of peppermint in a glass and pour over the pear. Chill for thirty minutes and garnish with half a cup of fresh blackcurrants.

Live Apple Sauce: Core and chop four apples and liquidise with enough apple juice to make a medium thick sauce. Add a dash of cinnamon or nutmeg and a little honey to sweeten. Serve immediately. (Add 125 g [4 oz] of chopped pecans for a nutritious all-fruit meal later in the day.)

The Vegetable Choice

I personally prefer pressed vegetable juices for breakfast. I especially like carrot with beetroot and some green leaves of dandelion, lettuce or spinach from the garden. If you have been used to a diet of convenience foods, however, you will probably want to introduce yourself slowly to the green foods. To start with, just add a leaf or two of a green vegetable to a glass of fresh fruit juice. Give yourself time to get used to the green flavours. As your body detoxifies you will not only find the greens easier to take; you are likely to end up loving them. When this happens you can use as much as 125 g (4 oz) of green leaf herbs and vegetables in a big glass of fresh fruit or vegetable juice.

Make a Great Salad

To most people a salad is a pleasant side dish used to set off a main course. All the salads here should, however, be used as the mainstay of an individual meal. They can be served on their own for lunch or dinner as a neutral meal (neither protein no carbohydrate-based). Or they can be combined with either a protein side-dish – nuts, fish, tofu, meat or eggs are good choices – to create a protein meal, or a starchy side dish – wholemeal bread, crispbreads, a baked potato, a vegetable rice dish, couscous or beans, such as kidney or butter beans – to create a starch meal. But remember, do not eat protein and starch at the same meal. Always choose the freshest vegetables and cut all the ingredients into bite-sized pieces.

You can make a deliciously quick and simple neutral salad by following this classic salad formula:

Take a grated root vegetable such as carrot or parsnip (not potato) and combine it with an equal amount of a leafy vegetable such as watercress, lamb's lettuce or Chinese leaf, and a bulb vegetable such as red or green pepper. Dress with olive oil, lemon juice, Worcester sauce and sea salt. Add either a protein element such as egg, or a carbohydrate element such as brown rice. Simple!

Here are a few more complex recipes to get your imagination working.

Green Glory (neutral)
Place 250 g (8 oz) of shredded Chinese leaves, 1 chopped green pepper, 3 tablespoons of finely chopped fresh mint, 4 sticks of chopped celery and 3 sliced spring onions in a bowl. Put 4 tablespoons of mayonnaise, 2 tablespoons of orange juice, the grated rind of half an orange, 2 tablespoons of fresh chopped parsley, 1 teaspoon of sea salt and 2 cloves of finely chopped garlic in a screw-topped jar, shake well and dress the salad. Add chopped boiled eggs or strips of vegetable omelette for a protein meal, or a baked potato to make a starch meal.

Root-is-Best Salad (neutral)
Mix together 2 finely grated turnips, 3 grated parsnips, 2 grated carrots, 3 chopped spring onions, half a green and half a red pepper (chopped) and 1 tablespoon of chopped savory or lovage. Pour the juice of 1 lemon over the salad. Toss and serve on a bed of grated Chinese leaves or lettuce. Serve with grated hard-boiled egg or a good-quality mayonnaise for protein or add toasted rye bread for a starch meal option.

Watercress Salad (neutral)

Mix together 3 handfuls of Cos lettuce, a bunch of chopped watercress, 4 chopped spring onions, 3 large courgettes (grated), 2 grated carrots and 4 quartered tomatoes. Make a light vinaigrette by blending 2 tablespoons of cider vinegar with 4 tablespoons of olive oil, half a teaspoon of Meaux mustard, half a teaspoon of tarragon, half a teaspoon of chervil, and half a teaspoon of sea salt. Add a small tin of tuna in brine or sprinkle 3–4 tablespoons of sunflower seeds over the salad for a tasty protein dish. Serve with buckwheat or steamed brown rice for a starch meal.

Tasty Toppings

The following protein-based dressings can be poured over salad or steamed vegetables to make a delicious lunch or dinner or used as a dip with crudités.

Nut Mayonnaise (protein)

In a blender or food processor blend 125 g (4 oz) of cashew nuts with a teacup of spring water, 2 cloves of chopped garlic, the juice of a lemon, 1 teaspoon of vegetable bouillon powder or tamari, and 3 finely chopped spring onions. Chill and serve.

Pink Tofu Dressing (protein)
Mix together 1 teacup of tofu, 2 tablespoons of tomato puree, 1 teaspoon of Meaux mustard, half a clove of finely chopped garlic and half a teaspoon of vegetable bouillon powder. Add 1 tablespoon of chopped shallots and mix again. Serve chilled. This will keep for about five days in the fridge.

Simple Soups

Avocado and Tomato (neutral)
Blend 6 ripe tomatoes, a ripe avocado, 2 finely chopped spring onions, ¼ teaspoon of dill seed, a pinch of cayenne, 300 ml (½ pint) of spring water, and 2 teaspoons of vegetable bouillon powder. Add 2 finely chopped tomatoes and a raw, finely chopped green pepper. Serve hot or cold, with wholemeal bread for a carbohydrate meal or topped with chopped, grilled bacon for a protein alternative.

Chilled Cucumber Soup (protein)
Blend a large, chopped cucumber with 2 cups soya milk and a

few ice cubes. Add 2 tablespoons vegetable bouillon powder and continue to blend. Then add 4 tablespoons chopped mint, blend briefly and serve immediately, topped with crushed poppy seeds.

Corn Soup (starch)
Wash 2 fresh corn cobs and cut the kernels off the cob. Mix the corn with 300 ml (½ pint) of warm spring water, 2 chopped spring onions, 1 teaspoon of olive oil and 1 teaspoon of vegetable bouillon powder or sea salt. Season with tahini (sesame seed paste) if desired, and blend until creamy.

Lunch or Dinner Recipes

Leave at least four to five hours between lunch and dinner for efficient digestion. Do not snack unless a meal is going to be delayed and it is more than four or five hours since you have eaten, in which case have a little fruit or a few raw vegetables. Most of these recipes are designed to feed four, but eat as much as you need, depending on how hungry you are. Take your time, chew thoroughly and stop as soon as you feel you have had enough.

Spicy Shish Kebab (neutral)

This is a delicious, marinated vegetable dish that you can grill or barbecue. Serve on a bed of brown rice that has been cooked in vegetable stock with a little chilli to make a satisfying meal or cut down on the vegetables and add 450 g (1 lb) of lamb or chicken chunks to the marinade and cook on the skewers for a delicious protein option.

Make a marinade in a large bowl by mixing together 1¼ teacups of olive oil, the juice of 3 lemons, 2 tablespoons of finely chopped parsley, ½ teaspoon of ground nutmeg, 1 tablespoon of chopped fresh basil and 1 teaspoon of dried oregano. Add 1 large aubergine cut into 3-cm (1¼-in) chunks, 10 halved fresh tomatoes, 24 large mushrooms, 1 red pepper, 1 green pepper, and 2 large red onions, all cut into chunks. Let it stand for three hours. Skewer the ingredients alternately and use the remaining marinade to baste them as they are grilled or barbecued.

Baked Leeks and Bacon (protein)

Slice 450 g (1 lb) leeks lengthways into very fine strips and then cut into 8-cm (3-in) lengths. Mix with 1 tablespoon of olive oil and bake in a hot oven for 10–15 minutes. Meanwhile, finely chop 125 g (4 oz) bacon and fry in its own fat. When the bacon is almost crispy, add 1 tablespoon of fresh chopped parsley, a splash of water and a pinch of salt and pepper. Pour over the leeks and serve. You can turn this into a carbohydrate meal by leaving out the bacon and replacing it with garlic croutons made by frying 125 g (4 oz) wholemeal bread cut into tiny squares in a little olive oil flavoured with garlic.

Polenta (starch)

This peasant dish made from cornmeal is delicious with a salad dressed in a spicy sauce. Heat ½ litre (¾ pint) of water in a kettle. Pour the boiling water into the saucepan over a teacupful of polenta cornmeal seasoned with a little sea salt. Stir until smooth and then cook very gently until all the liquid has been absorbed. Cool and drop by the spoonful onto a lightly oiled baking sheet. Grill until brown, turning once.

Super Stir-Fries

These attractive and marvellously quick meals are based on the Chinese principle of frying foods very quickly in a minute quantity of light oil to preserve texture and vitamins. They are easy to prepare. Simply chop all your ingredients finely so they cook in around three minutes. And don't be afraid to create your own combinations – just make sure that you don't mix carbohydrates and proteins in the same dish.

Sesame and Courgette Stir-Fry (protein)

Cut 250 g (8 oz) of courgettes, 8 sticks of celery and 250 g (8oz) of carrots into matchsticks. Heat 2 teaspoons of sesame or soya oil in a wok or frying pan. Add 125 g (4 oz) of sesame seeds and cook for 1–2 minutes until they start to brown. Add the vegetables and cook for another 2–3 minutes. Season with soy sauce or tamari and serve.

Ultra-High Stir-Fry (neutral)

Heat 2 teaspoons of soya oil or olive oil in a wok or large frying pan. Stir-fry 250 g (8 oz) of bean sprouts and a large, thinly-sliced red pepper for 2 minutes. Add soy sauce to taste, season with black pepper and serve. Add thin strips of pork or chicken to create a satisfying protein meal, or serve with fine noodles for a carbohydrate option.

Mangetout and Almond Stir-Fry (protein)

Top and tail 250 g (8 oz) of mangetout. Heat 2 teaspoons of soya oil or olive oil in a wok or large frying pan. When hot, add 50 g (2 oz) of blanched almonds and stir-fry for 3 minutes. Add the mangetout, 125 g (4 oz) of button mushrooms and soy sauce to taste. Serve immediately. Replace almonds with finely-sliced chicken or prawns if you like.

These are just a few suggestions. Make the most of what fruits and vegetables are freshest and in season and begin to experiment for yourself. Soon you will hardly have to think twice about whether a meal is protein, carbohydrate or neutral. Eating this way is a great insurance against contracting colds in the future as it not only provides your whole system with the nutrients it needs to keep healthy, it also helps to keep down the amount of toxic wastes that build up in your body causing you to get a cold in the first place. Winter will hold few fears for you. You may even have kicked colds for good.

RESOURCES

More from Leslie Kenton

Leslie lectures and teaches workshops throughout the world on health, authentic power, energy, creativity, shamanism, and spirituality. Two companies organise workshops for her in Britain: Bright Ideas provides workshops on health, energy and personal empowerment and books Leslie for lectures and individually-tailored seminars when these are requested. (For further ideas contact Bright Ideas: Telephone (in the UK) 08700 783783, or e-mail **LK@bright-idea.co.uk**) . Sacred Trust organises Leslie's residential and non-residential workshops on freedom, spirituality, creativity and shamanism. For further information contact The Sacred Trust, PO Box 603, Bath BA1 2ZU: Telephone 01225 852615, Fax 01225 858961.

Leslie's audio tapes including *10 Steps to a New You*, as well as her videos including *10 Day Clean Up Plan*, *Ageless Ageing*, *Lean Revolution*, *10 Day De-Stress Plan*, and *Cellulite Revolution*, can be ordered from QED Recording Services Ltd, Lancaster Road, New Barnet, Hertfordshire, EN4 8AS. Telephone 0181 441 7722, Fax 0181 441 0777. e-mail **Lesliekenton@qed-productions.com**

If you want to know about Leslie's personal appearances, forthcoming books, videos, workshops and projects please visit her website for the latest information: **http://www.qed-productions/lesliekenton.htm**

You can also write to her care of QED at the above address enclosing a stamped, self-addressed A4 sized envelope.

Suppliers

The Nutri Centre

7 Park Crescent, London W1N 3HE, Telephone 0171 436 5122, Fax 0171 436 5171
The Nutri Centre is on the lower ground floor of the Hale Clinic in London and has the finest selection of nutritional products and books on health under one roof in Britain – including all of Leslie Kenton's books – all available through a good mail-order service.

Higher Nature Limited

The Nutrition Centre, Burwash Common, East Sussex N19 7LX
Telephone 01435 882 880, Fax 01435 883 720
Higher Nature is the supplier of excellent nutritional supplements and some herbs. They sell good organic linseeds or flaxseeds.

Solgar Vitamins

Solgar House, Aldbury, Tring, Herts HP23 5PT, Telephone 01442 890 355, Fax 01442 890 366
An American company which produces good quality nutritional supplements and standardised single herbs and formulas under strict pharmaceutical standards of manufacture. Solgar products are available from top health-food stores, some chemists, and The Nutri Centre (above).

Phyto Products Ltd

Park Works, Park House, Mansfield Woodhouse, Notts NG19 8EF
Telephone 01623 644 334, Fax 01623 657 232
An excellent company originally set up to supply herbalists with high-quality herbs and plant products. They do not sell capsules but they now do some herbs in tablet form. Write to them for their price list. They have a minimum order of £20 (before VAT) plus carriage.

Simmonds Herbal Supplies

Freepost (BR1396), Hove, West Sussex, BN3 6BR, Telephone 01273 202 401, Fax 01273 705 120
This company has been supplying additive-free herbal aids to health practitioners in the UK and abroad since 1982. They also do a range of good-quality products for the general public, offering single herbs and mixtures as capsules, tinctures or extracts.

Bioforce (UK) Ltd

2 Brewster Place, Irvine, Ayrshire, Telephone 01563 851 177, Fax 01563 851 173
Suppliers of herbal extracts, tinctures, homeopathic remedies and natural self-care products and foods. They can be ordered by post but are often also available in good health-food stores and pharmacies carrying herbal products.

The Soil Association

The Organic Food & Farming Centre, 86 Coulson Street, Bristol BS1 5BB
Write to them for their regularly updated National Directory of Farm Shops and Box Schemes.

Organics Direct

1-7 Willow Street, London EC2A 4BH
Telephone 0171 729 2828. Or visit their website on **http://www.organicsdirect.com**. You can also order online.
Organics Direct offers a nationwide home delivery service of fresh vegetables and fruits, delicious breads, juices, sprouts, fresh soups, ready-made meals, snacks and baby foods. They even sell organic wines – all shipped to you within 24 hours.

Essential Oils: Top-quality aromatherapy products are available from *Sandra Day*, Ashley House, 185A Drake Street, Rochdale, Lancashire OL11 1E7: Telephone 01706 750302, Fax 01706 750 304. *The Fragrant Earth* Co Ltd, PO Box 182, Taunton, Somerset TA1 1YR: Telephone 01823 335 734, Fax 01823 322 566 do a good range as well.
Tisserand do an essential-oil diffuser that plugs in and fans the oils into the air. Contact *Tisserand Aromatherapy*, Newtown Road, Hove, Sussex BN3 7BA: Telephone 01273 325 666.

Flaxseeds/Linseeds: 'Linusit Gold' linseeds are available from *The Nutri Centre* (see above). Organic linseeds are also available from *Higher Nature* (see above). Keep them refrigerated.

Marigold Swiss Vegetable Bouillon Powder: This instant broth made from vegetables and sea salt comes in regular, low-salt, vegan and organic varieties. It is available from health-food stores, or direct from *Marigold Foods*, 102 Camley Street, London NW1 0PF: Telephone 0171 388 4515, Fax 0171 388 4516.

Water: Friends of the Earth have an excellent briefing sheet 'Drinking water: is it up to standard?' Contact *Friends of the Earth*, 26-28 Underwood Street, London N1 7JQ.

Water Filters: Contact *The Fresh Water Filter Company*, Carlton House, Aylmer Road, Leytonstone, London E11 3AD. Telephone 0181 558 7495, Fax 0181 556 9270.

Index